HEMOCHROMATOSIS MANAGEMENT DIET COOKBOOK

Balancing Nutrients: A Comprehensive Guide To Dietary Management: Optimal Health Through Dietary Balance:

DR. SHAYLA LEWIS

Table of Contents

DISCLAIMER

Write a brief complete Disclaimer for my diet cook book telling them that the author is not in any association with any company, business or individual and also this book is written by the authors knowledge and understanding

The information provided in this diet cookbook is based on the author's personal knowledge and understanding. The author is not affiliated with, endorsed by, or associated with any company, business, or individual. The recipes and dietary advice contained within this book are intended for informational purposes only. Readers should consult with a healthcare professional or a registered dietitian before making any significant changes to their diet or lifestyle. The author assumes no responsibility for any adverse effects that may result from the use or misuse of the information contained in this book.

CHAPTER ONE
What is hemochromatosis?

Hemochromatosis is sometimes referred to as an "iron overload disorder" since the predominant symptom is an abnormal accumulation of iron in the body. Excess iron is often retained in organs and tissues, causing damage and dysfunction. Hemochromatosis is classified into numerous kinds, the most prevalent of which is hereditary hemochromatosis, caused by mutations in the HFE gene. This gene generally regulates iron absorption from the food, but mutations can impair this process, resulting in excessive iron absorption.

Causes and Risk Factors:

The primary cause of hemochromatosis is hereditary, with mutations in certain genes, such as the HFE gene, accounting for the majority of cases. These genetic mutations are usually inherited in an autosomal recessive pattern, which means that a person must inherit two copies of the defective gene (one from each parent) to develop the disorder. However, not everyone with these genetic abnormalities develops hemochromatosis, as other factors such as diet and environment can impact the condition's onset and severity.

Hemochromatosis is known as a "silent" disease because symptoms may not develop until iron levels in the body are dangerously high. When symptoms do appear, they might range in intensity and include weariness, joint discomfort, abdominal pain, weakness, and skin coloring (bronze or greyish). Untreated hemochromatosis can progress to more serious problems, including liver cirrhosis, diabetes, heart disease, and arthritis.

Diet is critical in controlling hemochromatosis and avoiding problems caused by iron excess. While dietary iron is not the major cause of the illness, it can add to the body's total iron burden. Individuals with hemochromatosis are often advised to adopt a low-iron diet, which entails restricting the consumption of iron-rich foods such as red meat, liver, shellfish, and iron-fortified products. In addition to limiting dietary iron intake, additional dietary changes may be advised, such as avoiding vitamin C supplements and alcohol, both of which can increase iron absorption.

The Hemochromatosis Management Diet Cookbook's goals are as follows:

Education: The cookbook's goal is to educate people with hemochromatosis about the importance of food in treating their illness.

Readers can make informed decisions about their eating habits and lifestyles by learning everything they can about hemochromatosis, including its causes, symptoms, and nutritional recommendations.

Nutritional Guidance: The cookbook provides practical advice on how to adopt a hemochromatosis-friendly diet that is low in iron and good for overall health. It offers recipes and meal plans that aim to reduce iron intake while still providing balanced nutrition and enjoyable meals.

Recipe Development: The cookbook includes a wide range of low-iron recipes that are high in flavor, originality, and nutritional value. These recipes are intended to fit a variety of tastes, preferences, and dietary limitations, allowing people with hemochromatosis to follow their dietary requirements without feeling deprived or limited.

Meal Planning: In addition to recipes, the cookbook includes suggestions and tactics for meal planning and preparation to assist readers in incorporating hemochromatosis-friendly foods into their daily routines. By providing practical tools and resources, the cookbook enables people to take charge of their diet and manage their condition more successfully.

Promoting Wellness: In addition to regulating iron levels, the cookbook emphasizes the significance of overall wellness and making healthy lifestyle choices for those with hemochromatosis. It offers advice on exercise, stress management, and other lifestyle aspects that might affect health and well-being, allowing users to take a comprehensive approach to managing their illness.

Hemochromatosis is a disorder defined by excessive iron absorption, which can result in iron overload in the body. Nutrition is important in controlling this disorder because various dietary choices can worsen or alleviate symptoms. Individuals with hemochromatosis can maintain optimal health by knowing how different diets affect iron intake and metabolism.

How Diet Affects Hemochromatosis: Diet has a direct impact on how much iron the body absorbs. Foods high in heme iron, such as red meat and organ meats, greatly affect iron levels in hemochromatosis patients. Vitamin C, calcium, and tannins are among the dietary components that might either improve or hinder iron absorption. Individuals can effectively manage iron levels and limit the risk of hemochromatosis consequences by changing their eating habits.

Several critical nutrients are essential for controlling hemochromatosis symptoms. This includes:

Limit heme iron intake and get enough non-heme iron. Vitamin C promotes non-heme iron absorption and should be consumed in moderation.

Calcium inhibits iron absorption and can lower iron levels when ingested with meals.

Fruits, vegetables, and nuts contain antioxidants that can reduce oxidative stress caused by iron excess.

Omega-3 fatty acids are anti-inflammatory and may aid those with hemochromatosis.

Foods to Avoid and Embrace: People with hemochromatosis should avoid or limit their intake of foods high in heme iron, such as red meat, liver, and seafood. Additionally, processed foods fortified with iron should be consumed in moderation. Instead, include iron-rich plant foods like beans, lentils, tofu, and fortified cereals. Consume a diet high in fruits, vegetables, whole grains, and lean proteins to offer critical nutrients while limiting iron intake.

The importance of balance and moderation cannot be overstated when it comes to controlling hemochromatosis through nutrition. While it is vital to restrict iron-rich meals, it is also critical to consume enough amounts of other essential minerals to promote general health. Aim for a well-rounded diet that includes a range of nutrient-dense foods, but be cautious of portion sizes and frequency of consumption.

Plan meals with a variety of minerals, including non-heme iron sources and foods that limit iron absorption.

Eat plenty of fruits and vegetables to boost antioxidants and fiber.

Try alternative cooking methods like steaming or grilling to reduce the need for extra fats.

Prepare meals ahead of time to have nutritious options available all week long.

To optimize iron absorption and metabolism, stay hydrated, and limit alcohol consumption.

By incorporating these principles into your book, readers will get vital insights into the role of nutrition in hemochromatosis management, as well as practical suggestions for optimizing their dietary choices to enhance general health and well-being.

CHAPTER TWO

Low-carbohydrate diets can help with hemochromatosis.

Hemochromatosis is characterized by excessive iron absorption, resulting in iron overload in the body. High-carbohydrate diets, particularly those high in refined sugars and processed grains, might worsen this illness by increasing insulin resistance and iron absorption.

Low-carb diets improve blood sugar regulation and insulin sensitivity, perhaps reducing the symptoms of hemochromatosis. Individuals with hemochromatosis who reduce their carbohydrate intake might better manage their blood sugar levels and potentially reduce iron absorption, limiting future iron accumulation in the body.

Oxidative stress plays a significant role in the pathogenesis of hemochromatosis. Excessive iron levels in the body can produce free radicals, causing oxidative damage to cells, tissues, and organs.

Antioxidants contained in fruits, vegetables, nuts, seeds, and spices can neutralize free radicals and lower oxidative stress. Individuals with hemochromatosis can benefit from incorporating antioxidant-rich foods into their diet to help protect against the harmful consequences of iron overload.

Anti-inflammatory foods play an important role in symptom control.

Hemochromatosis can cause chronic inflammation, leading to consequences such as liver cirrhosis, arthritis, and heart disease.

Anti-inflammatory foods including fatty fish, leafy greens, berries, olive oil, and turmeric can lower inflammation in the body. Including these foods in one's diet can help decrease hemochromatosis symptoms while also improving overall health and well-being.

Creating wholesome and appetizing meals: Creating dishes with minimal carbs, high antioxidants, and anti-inflammatory properties demands imagination and culinary skills. Individuals with hemochromatosis can have rich and satisfying meals by integrating a variety of nutrient-dense products such as lean meats, healthy fats, colorful fruits and veggies, whole grains, and herbs and spices.

Experimenting with cooking techniques and flavor combinations can improve dish taste and appeal while maintaining nutritional content.

Prioritising low-carb, antioxidant-rich, and anti-inflammatory meals can provide long-term advantages for people with hemochromatosis. Dietary adjustments that control blood sugar levels, reduce oxidative stress, and reduce inflammation can help minimize issues associated with iron overload and enhance the overall quality of life.

Consistency and commitment to healthy eating habits are crucial for maximizing the long-term benefits of diet improvements. Individuals with hemochromatosis can improve their condition and promote maximum health and well-being for years to come by adjusting their diet and lifestyle.

In this chapter, we will look at the significant benefits that low-carb, antioxidant-rich, and anti-inflammatory diets provide for people with hemochromatosis. Each of these dietary components is critical to improving general health and alleviating hemochromatosis symptoms.

Low-carbohydrate diets:

Low-carbohydrate diets have received a lot of attention due to their ability to regulate blood sugar levels, help with weight loss, and improve cardiovascular health. For people with hemochromatosis, a low-carb diet can help prevent excessive iron absorption, lowering the risk of iron overload-related problems. Individuals who limit their consumption of refined carbs and sugars can better manage their insulin levels and reduce oxidative stress in the body.

Antioxidant-rich foods:

Antioxidants are vital chemicals that fight oxidative damage and inflammation in the body. Consuming a variety of antioxidant-rich foods, such as fruits, vegetables, nuts, and seeds, can help neutralize free radicals and protect cells from the harm caused by excessive iron accumulation. These meals not only promote overall health but also help to control hemochromatosis by lowering the risk of consequences including liver damage and joint pain.

Anti-inflammatory Diet:

Hemochromatosis is characterized by chronic inflammation, which can increase symptoms and problems. An anti-inflammatory diet focuses on whole foods that include anti-inflammatory characteristics, such as fatty fish, olive oil, leafy greens, and spices like turmeric and ginger. Individuals can assist reduce inflammation and enhance their general health by limiting their intake of processed foods and trans fats.

Understanding Diabetes Management in Hemochromatosis

This chapter delves into the complex interaction between hemochromatosis and diabetes, offering insight into the problems and options for effectively managing both disorders simultaneously.

The relationship between hemochromatosis and diabetes:

Hemochromatosis and diabetes frequently coexist, and studies show a bidirectional link between the two illnesses. Iron overload caused by hemochromatosis can affect insulin secretion and sensitivity, increasing the likelihood of developing diabetes or intensifying pre-existing diabetic symptoms.

Individuals with diabetes, on the other hand, may accumulate iron more quickly due to insulin resistance, complicating hemochromatosis therapy.

Strategies for managing blood sugar levels: Optimal blood sugar control is critical for those with hemochromatosis and diabetes. Lifestyle changes such as regular exercise, carbohydrate monitoring, and adherence to prescribed medication regimes can help stabilize blood glucose levels and reduce the risk of diabetes complications. Furthermore, combining dietary measures specific to both illnesses, such as eating low-glycemic index foods and practicing portion management, can help improve glycemic control and general health.

The importance of glycemic control: Maintaining proper glycemic management is critical for preserving organ function and lowering the risk of long-term consequences from diabetes and hemochromatosis. Uncontrolled blood sugar levels can have major health effects, such as heart disease, neuropathy, and kidney damage.

Individuals who persistently monitor blood glucose levels and use proactive methods to treat insulin resistance and iron overload can reduce the negative impacts of both disorders and enhance their quality of life.

Include Diabetic-Friendly Foods in Your Diet: Adopting a diabetic-friendly diet is critical for regulating blood sugar levels and improving overall health in those with hemochromatosis and diabetes. Eating nutrient-dense foods including lean proteins, whole grains, fruits, and vegetables can help manage insulin levels and improve metabolic function. Furthermore, implementing diabetic-friendly swaps and substitutes, such as utilizing natural sweeteners instead of refined sugars and choosing complex carbohydrates over simple sugars, can help with blood sugar management while maintaining taste and satisfaction.

Balancing Nutritional Needs in Both Conditions:

Finding the correct balance between the dietary needs of hemochromatosis and diabetes is critical for getting the best health outcomes. Individuals can modify their diet to fit the particular needs of both illnesses by prioritizing nutrient-dense, whole foods while also paying attention to portion sizes and macronutrient composition.

Consulting with healthcare specialists, such as certified dietitians or nutritionists, can provide personalized direction and support as you navigate the challenges of controlling hemochromatosis and diabetes with food.

CHAPTER THREE

Understanding the Risks of Iron Overload: Iron overload, also known as hemochromatosis, is a disorder in which the body absorbs and accumulates an excessive amount of iron.

This excess iron can progressively accumulate in multiple organs such as the liver, heart, pancreas, and joints, causing major health consequences if left untreated.

Common consequences of iron overload include liver damage (cirrhosis), diabetes, heart disease, arthritis, and an increased risk of some malignancies. Individuals with hemochromatosis must understand these dangers to take proactive actions toward appropriate disease management.

Monitoring Iron and Ferritin Levels: Individuals with hemochromatosis must regularly check their iron and ferritin levels to assess the progression of their condition and make informed treatment and dietary decisions. Serum iron, transferrin saturation, and serum ferritin are all blood tests that can be used to measure iron levels. Ferritin is a protein that accumulates iron in the body; high ferritin levels suggest excessive iron accumulation. Monitoring these levels enables healthcare practitioners to determine the severity of iron overload and modify treatment approaches accordingly.

Diet and lifestyle changes can help manage hemochromatosis and prevent problems caused by iron overload.

Important dietary changes include lowering your intake of iron-rich foods such as red meat, liver, seafood, and iron-fortified meals. Furthermore, it is advisable to avoid vitamin C supplements and heavy alcohol usage, as these can improve iron absorption. A balanced diet rich in fruits, vegetables, whole grains, and lean proteins will help you maintain good health while limiting your iron intake. Regular exercise, maintaining a healthy weight, and abstaining from tobacco use are all crucial lifestyle choices for hemochromatosis patients.

Regular medical check-ups and blood tests are critical components of hemochromatosis care because they help monitor iron levels, assess liver function, and screen for potential consequences.

Healthcare practitioners may propose routine blood tests to assess serum iron, transferrin saturation, serum ferritin, liver enzymes, and other pertinent markers. These check-ups enable early detection of changes in iron levels or liver function, allowing for fast intervention and treatment plan adjustments as needed. Consistent monitoring helps to avoid the advancement of hemochromatosis and lowers the risk of significant consequences.

 Living with hemochromatosis can be difficult, both physically and mentally. Seeking help from healthcare specialists, such as primary care physicians, hematologists, hepatologists, and registered dietitians, is critical for the condition's overall management.

These specialists can provide personalized advice, treatment alternatives, and ongoing monitoring to improve health outcomes. Furthermore, interacting with support groups and online networks for hemochromatosis patients can provide significant emotional support, practical advice, and a feeling of community.

CHAPTER FOUR

Is it possible to heal hemochromatosis by food alone?

Hemochromatosis, specifically hereditary hemochromatosis (HH), is a genetic disorder that causes excessive absorption of dietary iron, resulting in iron overload in the body. While nutrition can help manage hemochromatosis, it cannot cure it completely. The primary treatment for hemochromatosis is phlebotomy (blood removal) to lower iron levels in the body. A well-planned diet, on the other hand, can supplement medical treatment by regulating iron intake and lowering the risk of hemochromatosis consequences.

Is it safe to donate blood with hemochromatosis?

Yes, donating blood is frequently suggested as a treatment for people with hemochromatosis. Regular blood donations, also known as phlebotomy or therapeutic phlebotomy, are an efficient method for lowering iron levels in the body. Individuals suffering from hemochromatosis can reduce their risk of iron overload-related problems such as liver damage, joint discomfort, and weariness by donating blood. Individuals with hemochromatosis should speak with their healthcare professional to identify the most appropriate frequency of blood donations based on their condition and iron levels.

Can vitamins assist with hemochromatosis?
While certain supplements may help manage hemochromatosis, they should be used with caution and under the supervision of a

healthcare expert. Iron supplements, in particular, should be avoided by people who have hemochromatosis since they can worsen iron excess. However, some people with hemochromatosis may need to take additional supplements to address deficits produced by the disorder or its complications, such as vitamin C to improve iron excretion or vitamin D to promote bone health. Individuals with hemochromatosis should consult with their healthcare professional to identify the best supplementation program based on their specific needs and iron status.

What are the possible complications of hemochromatosis?

Untreated hemochromatosis can cause a variety of consequences, most notably the accumulation of excess iron in the body's tissues and organs.

Liver injury (cirrhosis or hepatocellular cancer)

Joint discomfort and arthritis.

Diabetes mellitus.

Heart conditions (cardiomyopathy, arrhythmias)

Skin discoloration (bronze or greyish color)

Thyroid problems.

Sexual dysfunction and infertility.

How may family members be assessed for hemochromatosis risk?

Because hemochromatosis is predominantly a genetic disorder, it is critical to test family members for the disease, particularly if a close relative has been diagnosed. Typically, genetic testing is used to find mutations in the HFE gene, which is linked to hereditary hemochromatosis.

Family members of people with hemochromatosis should undergo genetic testing if they are concerned about their risk or have signs of iron excess.

Furthermore, healthcare experts may propose screening for iron overload in family members of hemochromatosis patients using blood tests such as serum ferritin levels to determine their iron status. Early discovery through screening can lead to timely intervention and preventative measures, lowering the risk of hemochromatosis consequences.

By thoroughly answering these common concerns and misconceptions, your readers will obtain a better understanding of hemochromatosis and its treatment, allowing them to make more educated decisions regarding their health and well-being.

Breakfast alternatives to start the day:
Iron-conscious Smoothie: Use antioxidant-rich components such as spinach, kale, berries, and chia seeds. To increase iron absorption, add vitamin C-rich fruits such as oranges or strawberries.

Quinoa Breakfast Bowl: Quinoa is high in protein and fiber, and low in iron. To add flavor and nutrients, top with nuts, seeds, and fresh fruits.

Egg White Omelette: Egg whites are a protein-rich food with low iron content. Fill your omelet with vegetables like peppers, onions, and mushrooms to receive more vitamins and minerals.

Muesli with Almond Milk: Oats are naturally low in iron but high in fiber. Cook them with almond milk for a creamy texture, then top with nuts and fruits for extra nutrition.

Salads and soups that are satisfying for lunch

Spinach and Strawberry Salad: Spinach is low in iron, while strawberries provide flavor and vitamin C. Add grilled chicken or tofu for protein.

Quinoa Salad with Avocado: Quinoa is a complete protein with low iron. Combine it with chopped avocado, cherry tomatoes, cucumber, and a lemon vinaigrette for a delicious supper.

Minestrone Soup: This hearty and healthful soup is full of veggies and legumes. To add extra nutrition, use low-sodium broth and leafy greens such as kale or Swiss chard.

Tuna Salad with Leafy Greens: Tuna is a protein-rich food with low iron content. Serve it over a bed of mixed greens with olive oil and lemon dressing.

Delicious main meals for dinner:
Salmon with Roasted Vegetables: Salmon is high in omega-3 fatty acids but low in iron.

For a well-balanced supper, serve with roasted veggies such as broccoli, bell peppers, and carrots.

Turkey Chilli: Lean ground turkey is a healthier alternative to beef and has less iron. Fill your chili with beans, tomatoes, onions, and spices for a tasty meal.

Stir-fried Tofu with Vegetables: Tofu, a plant-based protein, is naturally low in iron. Stir-fry it with a variety of colorful veggies and a ginger-garlic sauce for a delicious supper.

Grilled Chicken with Quinoa Pilaf: Chicken breasts are lean and low in iron. For a wholesome evening, serve it with vegetable and herb-infused quinoa pilaf.

Healthy food that fulfills cravings:
Vegetable Sticks with Hummus: Crunchy vegetables like carrots, cucumber, and bell peppers are high in fiber and low in iron. Pair

them with homemade hummus for a filling snack.

Greek Yoghurt Parfait: Greek yogurt is rich in protein but low in iron. For a healthful and tasty treat, top it with fresh fruits, nuts, and a drizzle of honey.

Edamame is a high-protein, low-iron bean. Boil them and season with sea salt for a quick and healthy snack.

Apple slices with almond butter: Apples are low in iron but high in fiber. Spread almond butter on apple slices for a sweet and filling treat.

Indulgent but healthful desserts:
Dark Chocolate Avocado Mousse: Avocado contributes creaminess and healthful fats to this delectable dessert, and dark chocolate contains antioxidants. Sweeten with a small amount of honey or maple syrup.

Berry Chia Seed Pudding: Chia seeds are high in fibre, but low in iron. Mix them with your favorite fruit and almond milk, then set aside overnight for a delicious and nutritious custard.

Banana Nice Cream: Blend frozen bananas until smooth for a guilt-free ice cream substitute. For added flavor, mix it with some chocolate powder or peanut butter.

Baked Apples with Cinnamon: Core the apples and fill them with oats, cinnamon, and honey. Bake till soft for a warm and satisfying dessert choice.

These meals not only meet the nutritional demands of people with hemochromatosis, but they also emphasize flavor and nutrition, making mealtime fun and rewarding.

Incorporating Physical Activity into Your Routine: Physical activity is essential for effectively controlling hemochromatosis. Regular exercise promotes a healthy body weight, improves insulin sensitivity, and reduces inflammation. In your book, you can describe a variety of workouts appropriate for people with hemochromatosis, such as low-impact activities like walking, swimming, and cycling. You may also offer advice on how to progressively increase physical activity while taking into account individual limitations and preferences.

CHAPTER FIVE

Managing Stress and Prioritising Self-Care: Stress management is critical for general health, particularly for people with hemochromatosis. Chronic stress can worsen symptoms and raise the risk of problems. In your book, look at stress-reduction approaches like mindfulness meditation, deep breathing exercises, and relaxation techniques. Encourage readers to prioritize self-care activities like hobbies, spending time in nature, and practicing gratitude to improve their mental and emotional well-being.

Importance of Adequate Hydration: Proper hydration is critical for those with hemochromatosis because it promotes liver function and prevents dehydration, which is a significant worry for those undergoing therapeutic phlebotomy. In your book, stress the need to drink water throughout the day and include practical methods for improving water intake, such as carrying a reusable water bottle, flavoring water with fruits or herbs, and setting reminders to drink water at regular intervals.

Sleep Hygiene Tips for Better Rest: Quality sleep is essential for controlling hemochromatosis since it boosts general health and immunological function. Individuals with hemochromatosis may develop sleep difficulties as a result of symptoms such as joint discomfort, exhaustion, or restless leg syndrome. In your book, include sleep hygiene suggestions such as sticking to a consistent sleep schedule, developing a soothing evening routine, optimizing the sleep environment, and avoiding stimulants like caffeine and electronic devices before bedtime.

Salmon and Avocado Wrap

Grilled salmon flakes wrapped in a whole-grain tortilla with avocado, lettuce, and tomatoes.

Vegetable Stir-Fry with Tofu

Stir-fry broccoli, bell peppers, carrots, and snap peas with tofu cubes in light soy sauce.

Chicken and Vegetable Skewers

Marinate chicken breast chunks with olive oil, garlic, lemon juice, and herbs. Thread cherry tomatoes, mushrooms, and zucchini onto skewers and grill until well cooked.

Quinoa Stuffed Bell Peppers

Fill halved bell peppers with cooked quinoa, black beans, corn, chopped tomatoes, and spices. Bake until soft.

Turkey and Spinach Meatballs

Combine ground turkey, spinach, garlic, breadcrumbs, and egg. Roll into meatballs and bake until golden brown.

Mediterranean Lentil Soup

Simmered lentils with onions, carrots, celery, diced tomatoes, and Mediterranean spices (cumin, coriander, and paprika).

Baked Cod with Herb Crust

Top cod fillets with breadcrumbs, parsley, lemon zest, and garlic, and bake until crispy and flaky.

Roasted vegetable quiche

Combine roasted vegetables like zucchini, bell peppers, and onions with beaten eggs. Pour into a pie crust and bake until set.

Greek Yoghurt Parfait.

Top Greek yogurt with fresh berries, sliced bananas, and nuts or granola for crunch.

Now for a 30-day meal plan:

Week 1:

Breakfast: Greek yogurt parfait.

Lunch: Quinoa salad with lemon-tahini dressing.

Dinner: Baked cod with herb crust, steamed broccoli, and quinoa.

Week 2:

Breakfast: Whole-grain toast with avocado and sliced tomatoes.

Lunch: Mediterranean lentil soup with a mixed green salad.

Dinner: Vegetable stir-fry with tofu, served with brown rice

Week 3:

Breakfast: Spinach and Feta Omelette.

Lunch: Turkey and spinach meatballs served with roasted sweet potatoes and green beans.

Dinner: Salmon and avocado wrap, with carrot sticks on the side.

Week 4:

Breakfast: Berry smoothie with spinach, mixed berries, banana, and almond milk.

Lunch: Quinoa-stuffed bell peppers served with mixed greens.

Dinner: Chicken and veggie skewers with quinoa salad.

Remember to alter portion sizes to meet your unique nutritional needs and tastes, and always get personalized dietary advice from a healthcare expert.

To summarise, "The Hemochromatosis Management Diet Cookbook" seeks to provide persons diagnosed with hemochromatosis with delicious and healthy dishes suited to their specific dietary needs. Hemochromatosis, a disorder characterized by high iron absorption, needs cautious dietary choices to properly manage iron levels while maintaining general health.

Throughout this cookbook, we've looked at a variety of savory and satisfying meals that use low-iron sources while emphasizing key nutrients and culinary satisfaction. From vivid salads overflowing with fresh vegetables to protein-packed mains containing lean meats and plant-based alternatives, each recipe has been deliberately designed to aid in hemochromatosis management without sacrificing flavor or nutritional content.

In addition to presenting a varied range of dishes, this cookbook is a useful resource for people dealing with hemochromatosis. By providing comprehensive advice on food selection, cooking techniques, and meal planning strategies, readers can be confident in their capacity to make informed nutritional choices that correspond with their health goals.

Furthermore, the 30-day meal plan provided in this book provides a methodical strategy to integrate these hemochromatosis-friendly foods into daily life, simplifying meal preparation while providing a balanced and diverse diet.

Finally, "The Hemochromatosis Management Diet Cookbook" is more than simply a collection of recipes; it's an invaluable resource for anyone looking to take charge of their health and well-being via conscious and tasty eating. Readers can enhance their health and quality of life by adopting a nutrient-dense diet and being cautious of iron content when treating their hemochromatosis condition.

THE END

www.ingramcontent.com/pod-product-compliance
Lightning Source LLC
Chambersburg PA
CBHW071217260726
48653CB00041B/893